KNOWLEDGE GUIDE TO DUPUYTREN'S CONTRACTURE

Comprehensive Manual To Symptoms, Treatments, And Preventative Care For Hand Health And Mobility

DR. AARON BRANUM

Copyright © 2024 BY DR. AARON BRANUM

All rights reserved. Except for brief quotations embodied in critical reviews and certain other noncommercial uses permitted by copyright law, no part of this publication may be reproduced, distributed, or transmitted in any form or by any means, Including photocopying, recording, or other electronic or mechanical methods, without the prior written permission of the publisher.

Disclaimer:

The data in this book, is solely meant to be informative and instructional.

This book is not intended to replace expert medical advice, diagnosis, or care. No medical, health, or other professional services are offered by the author, publisher, or any affiliated parties

Individual outcomes may differ in the practice of these therapies, which entail a variety of approaches and methodologies.

A one-on-one session with a trained or certified healthcare professional is still preferable. It is best to consult a trained healthcare provider before making any decisions regarding your health.

The author of this book is not affiliated with any specific website, product, or organization related to any of these therapies.

All reasonable measures have been taken by the author and publisher to guarantee the authenticity and dependability of the material contained in this book

Contents

CHAPTER ONE 13
  ANATOMY AND RESOURCES 13
    How The Hand Is Anatomized 13
    What Leads To The Contracture Of Dupuytren? 14
    Risk Elements Linked To The Illness 14
    Biological Propensity 15
    Environmental Elements That Could Be Involved 15

CHAPTER TWO 17
  DIAGNOSIS 17
    A Medical Professional's Physical Examination 17
    Recognizing The Condition's Severity 18
    The Value Of Quickly Seeking Medical Advice 19

CHAPTER THREE 21
  OPTIONS FOR TREATMENT 21
    Methods Of Non-Surgical Treatment 21
    Drugs And Injectables 22

Exercises And Physical Therapy...............23

Procedures Surgical...............................24

Alternative Medicines And Their Performance 25

CHAPTER FOUR 27

GETTING READY FOR SURGERY 27

Speaking With An Expert........................27

Examinations And Tests Prior To Surgery .28

Comprehending The Surgical Process.......28

The Dangers And Issues Related To Surgery 29

Getting Physically And Mentally Ready For The Procedure 30

Procedures In Surgery 31

CHAPTER FIVE 35

CARE AFTER POSTOPERATION 35

Instructions For Immediate Post-Surgery Care..35

Hand Therapy And Rehabilitation............36

Handling Soreness And Unease 37

Keeping Complications Like Infection And Recurrence At Bay 38

  Extended Monitoring And Follow-Up 39

CHAPTER SIX 41

  REPAY AND RESUMMATION 41

  Timetable For Recuperation 41

  Improvement In Hand Function Gradually 43

  The Value Of Following Rehabilitation Exercises 44

  Picking Up Daily Tasks And Work 45

  Psychological Assistance Throughout The Healing Process 47

CHAPTER SEVEN 49

  MANAGING DUPUYTREN'S CONTRACTURE: COPING MECHANISMS 49

  Managing Physical Restrictions 49

  Asking Friends And Family For Support 50

  Taking Part In Online Communities And Support Groups 50

  Tools And Adaptive Devices For Everyday Tasks 51

  Adopting A Positive Attitude And Mindset .52

CHAPTER EIGHT 55
FAQS AND REGULAR QUESTIONS 55
Is It Possible To Avoid Dupuytren's Contracture? 55

Does Dupuytren's Contracture Run In Families? 57

What Is The Likelihood Of A Recurrence Following Surgery? 58

Can Altering One's Lifestyle Aid In Managing The Illness? 59

Sustaining An Appropriate Weight: 60

CONCERNING THIS BOOK

The "Knowledge Guide to Dupuytren's Contracture" is an invaluable resource for anyone coping with this difficult hand condition, offering empowerment and understanding. The primary goal of the book is to solve the puzzle of Dupuytren's Contracture by providing a thorough examination that covers everything from the anatomical foundations to the subtleties of diagnostic and treatment options.

The book begins with an explanation of Dupuytren's Contracture, laying the groundwork for a thorough examination of its nuances. Through a voyage of understanding, readers come to understand the nature of this illness, how common it is, and the warning signs that need to be taken seriously. Most importantly, it highlights how important early detection is and how prompt action can slow the disease's course and improve treatment results.

By delving into anatomy and etiology, the book explains the triggers behind Dupuytren's Contracture and reveals the intricate workings of the hand. Every aspect is carefully broken down, from environmental causes to genetic predispositions, equipping readers with the information to identify their personal risk factors.

The diagnosis section acts as a compass, guiding readers through the maze of medical evaluations that are essential for determining a proper prognosis. Readers are able to assess the severity of their ailment through the use of both modern imaging techniques and physical assessments, which emphasizes the need for prompt expert guidance.

A wide range of methods for treatment are available, from non-surgical therapies to the complexities of surgical operations. With a comprehensive comprehension of drug regimes, physical therapy, and surgical consultations, readers may confidently and clearly manage their treatment journey.

An important chapter that outlines the procedures for preparedness and well-informed decision-making is Surgery Preparation. Through medical consultations and mental and physical preparations, readers are equipped to approach surgery with a combination of resilience and practicality.

The section on surgical procedures provides readers with the necessary knowledge to make informed judgments about treatment by clarifying the nuances of fasciotomy and fasciectomy. Postoperative care is a ray of hope, providing direction on how to travel the path to recovery with diligence and resolve.

The story of recovery and rehabilitation is one of tenacity; it outlines the course of recovery and highlights the significance of following rehabilitation guidelines. Coping mechanisms surface as a lifeline during the ups and downs of recovery, providing comfort and encouragement through mental and physical hardships.

Finally, the book's conclusion in FAQs and frequently asked questions provides a lifeline of certainty by skillfully and sympathetically answering any last-minute questions and reservations. Readers find comfort in a wealth of information, enabling them to regain control over their health and well-being through preventative actions and support options.

Beyond the realm of a simple manual, the "Knowledge Guide to Dupuytren's Contracture" is a monument to the human spirit, providing direction, comfort, and hope to individuals attempting to make their way through the maze-like passages of Dupuytren's Contracture.

CHAPTER ONE

ANATOMY AND RESOURCES

How The Hand Is Anatomized

Gaining an understanding of the complex anatomy of the hand is crucial to understanding Dupuytren's contracture.

The hand is a miracle of nature, with bones, muscles, ligaments, tendons, and nerves all cooperating to carry out a variety of tasks.

The palm, which is where the disease mainly shows itself, is at the center of this intricate arrangement.

The network of tissues that makes up the palm includes the palmar fascia, which is essential for hand flexibility and movement.

What Leads To The Contracture Of Dupuytren?

The thick band of tissue in the palm called the palmar fascia can thicken and tighten unnaturally over time, resulting in Dupuytren's contracture.

The fingers bend inward towards the palm as a result of this tightness, limiting their range of motion. Although the precise cause of Dupuytren's contracture is still unknown, a number of factors are thought to play a role in its development.

Risk Elements Linked To The Illness

Dupuytren's contracture is more likely to occur due to a number of causes. Individuals can determine their susceptibility to the disorder and, if necessary, take preventive action by being aware of these risk factors.

Biological Propensity

Dupuytren's contracture is largely genetically based, and the ailment frequently runs in families. You may be more susceptible to developing Dupuytren's contracture if you have a close family who has had it, such as a parent or sibling. Scholars have detected specific genetic markers linked to a heightened likelihood of the disorder, underscoring the hereditary aspect of Dupuytren's contracture.

Environmental Elements That Could Be Involved

Dupuytren's contracture develops as a result of both environmental and genetic causes, though genetics plays a significant impact.

These variables could be things like work-related exposures, personal behaviors, and outside influences. People who perform heavy manual labor or participate in repetitive hand movements, for instance, may be more susceptible to developing the illness. Additionally, there is evidence linking an increased occurrence of Dupuytren's contracture to specific health disorders, including drinking and diabetes.

By changing their lifestyle and taking preventative action, people can reduce their risk by being aware of certain environmental influences.

CHAPTER TWO

DIAGNOSIS

A Medical Professional's Physical Examination

A physical examination performed by a healthcare provider is an essential first step in identifying Dupuytren's contracture.

The physician will carefully examine the affected hand or hands during this examination to look for any indications of contractures, nodules, or thickened or hardened tissue. Additionally, they will assess the fingers' and palms' range of motion, searching for any restrictions or abnormalities.

The healthcare professional can obtain crucial data regarding the scope and gravity of the ailment through this practical evaluation.

Imaging Tests Like Ultrasound In certain situations, medical professionals may use imaging tests like ultrasound to help diagnose Dupuytren's contracture. With the help of ultrasound imaging, medical experts can obtain precise images of the hand's structures and more easily identify any anomalies, such as thickening tissue or nodules.

With the aid of this diagnostic instrument, Dupuytren's contracture can be identified and its severity can be evaluated. Since ultrasound imaging is non-invasive and usually painless, it is an important diagnostic tool.

Recognizing The Condition's Severity

Knowing the degree of Dupuytren's contracture is crucial once the problem has been diagnosed. Individual differences in intensity can be observed, ranging from mild symptoms that have little effect on hand function to more severe cases where the contracture severely restricts movement and functionality. To evaluate the severity of the problem, medical professionals will look at a variety of variables, such as the quantity and size of nodules, the extent of contracture, and the effect on hand function. Healthcare practitioners can use this information to create individualized management plans for each patient and to guide treatment decisions.

The Value Of Quickly Seeking Medical Advice

Those who think they may develop Dupuytren's contracture or who are exhibiting signs like thickening of the palm or trouble straightening fingers should consult a doctor right once. Hand function can be preserved and the condition's progression can be halted with early identification and treatment.

People who seek medical advice as soon as possible can be given an accurate diagnosis, informed about their options for therapy, and started on the right management techniques to keep their hands mobile and functional.

Delaying getting a medical evaluation could cause Dupuytren's contracture to worsen and cause problems in the future.

For this reason, it's critical to give obtaining medical advice first priority as soon as Dupuytren's contracture symptoms appear in order to guarantee prompt action and the best possible results.

CHAPTER THREE

OPTIONS FOR TREATMENT

Individual differences exist in the severity and course of Dupuytren's contracture. Treatment choices therefore can change depending on a patient's unique situation. We'll look at all of the various treatment choices here, including non-surgical methods, surgical procedures, and alternative therapies.

Methods Of Non-Surgical Treatment

When Dupuytren's contracture is first developing or when the symptoms are not severe, non-surgical treatments are frequently taken into consideration. Using orthotic equipment, like braces or splints, to assist extend and straighten the afflicted fingers is one popular method. These devices can help slow down the progression of contractures and are usually worn at night.

Injectable collagenase is another non-surgical alternative. The enzyme collagenase has the ability to break down the collagen accumulation that is causing the contracture. After the injection is made directly into the damaged tissue, the enzyme gradually breaks down the extra collagen over the course of a few days, allowing the finger to straighten.

Drugs And Injectables

Other drugs could be recommended in addition to collagenase injections to assist in controlling symptoms or stop Dupuytren's contracture from getting worse.

One such drug is called Xiaflex, and it's a refined collagenase supplement that's authorized to treat Dupuytren's contracture. By dissolving extra collagen, Xiaflex is injected directly into the damaged tissue and functions similarly to collagenase injections.

Injections of corticosteroids can also be used to lessen inflammation and ease the symptoms of Dupuytren's contracture. When nodules or cords are causing discomfort, these injections can help reduce pain and increase the range of motion in the afflicted fingers.

Exercises And Physical Therapy

Dupuytren's contracture can be effectively managed with physical therapy and focused exercises, particularly when combined with other forms of treatment.

A physical therapist might offer advice on certain exercises intended to increase the afflicted fingers' range of motion and flexibility. These finger-maintenance activities could involve light stretching, massages, and gripping drills.

Dupuytren's contracture-related discomfort and stiffness may also be lessened with the use of hand therapy methods like heat or ultrasound therapy.

These techniques can enhance tissue repair and blood flow to the injured area, which will ultimately improve hand function as a whole.

Procedures Surgical

Surgical intervention may be required if non-surgical therapy is unable to sufficiently address symptoms or if contractures worsen. In order to improve finger extension, Dupuytren's contracture surgery usually entails either excising the thicker tissue (fasciectomy) or severing the contracted cords (fasciotomy).

Open surgery, percutaneous needle fasciotomy, and less invasive procedures like needle aponeurotomy are among the surgical options that are available.

The patient's general health status, the severity of the contracture, and the existence of complications all influence the technique that is chosen.

Alternative Medicines And Their Performance

Dupuytren's contracture is primarily managed with traditional medical therapy; however, some patients may choose to add complementary or alternative therapies to their regimen.

These could be herbal medicines, massage therapy, acupuncture, or dietary supplements with the promise of reducing inflammation or improving collagen.

But before attempting any alternative remedies, it's crucial to talk about them with a healthcare professional and approach them cautiously.

Although there is a lack of scientific evidence to support the usefulness of alternative therapies for Dupuytren's contracture, some individuals may experience relief from symptoms or an improvement in hand function with them.

Prioritizing evidence-based treatments is essential, as is speaking with a healthcare provider to create a thorough treatment plan that is customized to each patient's requirements and preferences.

CHAPTER FOUR

GETTING READY FOR SURGERY

Speaking With An Expert

It's imperative to arrange a consultation with a specialist, usually an orthopedic or hand surgeon with experience treating Dupuytren's contracture, prior to undergoing surgery for the ailment.

The expert will examine your hand in great detail during the appointment and go over your medical history, including any prior operations or treatments for Dupuytren's contracture.

You can address any worries you may have regarding the procedure and ask questions at this time.

Examinations And Tests Prior To Surgery

Your surgeon may request a number of pre-operative tests and evaluations in order to make sure you're in good health and to collect data that will help direct the surgical strategy.

Blood tests, imaging procedures like MRIs and X-rays, and potentially an electrocardiogram (ECG) to evaluate heart function are some examples of these tests.

Further examinations or consultations with other medical professionals might be required, contingent on your general health status and any current medical issues.

Comprehending The Surgical Process

It is critical that you comprehend the surgical treatment that will be performed to treat Dupuytren's contracture. The specifics of the surgery, such as the kind of anesthetic to be utilized, the site of the incision, and the methods to be utilized in order to release the contracted tissue in your hand, will be covered by your specialist. They will also go over the anticipated results of the procedure, such as enhanced hand function and any possible drawbacks or hazards.

The Dangers And Issues Related To Surgery

Surgery to treat Dupuytren's contracture entails some risks and possible complications, just like any other surgical operation. It's important to be aware of these as you get ready for the procedure; your specialist will go over them with you at the appointment. Infection, hemorrhage, nerve injury, and post-operative hand stiffness or weakening are common complications. By applying sterile techniques and carefully designing the surgical strategy based on your unique anatomy and condition, your specialist will take precautions to minimize these risks.

Getting Physically And Mentally Ready For The Procedure

Making the necessary physical and emotional preparations for surgery is a crucial step in the procedure. Asking questions, educating yourself about the process, and sharing any worries with your loved ones or your healthcare staff can all help you mentally prepare for the treatment. Additionally, lowering anxiety before the procedure might be achieved by engaging in mindfulness or relaxation exercises.

Physically, in the days or weeks preceding surgery, your doctor could give you specific recommendations to follow. This could include advice on which medications to avoid, dietary recommendations, and how to take care of your hands both before and after the treatment. To increase the likelihood of a positive result and reduce the possibility of problems, it is imperative that you carefully follow these directions. In order to lower the chance of problems, it's also critical to properly manage any underlying medical disorders you may have, such as diabetes or high blood pressure, in the days before surgery.

Procedures In Surgery

There are various surgical techniques available for treating Dupuytren's contracture, each with pros and cons of their own. Having a thorough understanding of these processes will enable you to choose the one that might be appropriate for your circumstances.

Comparing Fasciotomy with Fasciectomy: What's the Difference?

Two popular surgical techniques for treating Dupuytren's contracture are fasciotomy and fasciectomy; however, they vary in technique and degree of tissue removal.

Percutaneous Fasciotomy with Needle

A needle is used in percutaneous needle fasciotomy (PNF), a minimally invasive treatment, to break up the thickened tissue in the hand's palm. For patients who are not candidates for more involved surgery or for those with early-stage Dupuytren's contracture, this technique is frequently advised.

Fasciotomy Open

An incision is made in the palm of the hand during an open fasciotomy treatment to access and loosen the tight bands of tissue that are causing the contracture. In contrast to fasciectomy, which involves the removal of tissue, fasciotomy is a less intrusive procedure that requires a shorter recovery period.

Restricted Fasciectomy

A limited fasciectomy preserves as much of the healthy tissue as feasible while removing only the diseased tissue that caused the contracture. Patients who wish to maintain as much hand function as possible but have mild to severe Dupuytren's contracture are generally advised to have this treatment.

Whole Face Excision and Its Modifications

A more involved surgical technique called a full fasciectomy involves the removal of all diseased tissue that is the source of the contracture. Variations of this operation, including dermofasciectomy, in which the overlaying skin is also removed, may be carried out, depending on the severity of the contracture and the unique circumstances of the patient.

The optimal surgical option for you will depend on a number of criteria, including the severity of your condition, your general health, and your personal preferences. Each surgical method for Dupuytren's contracture has advantages and disadvantages of its own. To choose the best course of action for you, it's crucial to go over your options with your healthcare professional.

CHAPTER FIVE

CARE AFTER POSTOPERATION

Instructions For Immediate Post-Surgery Care

It's critical to follow the post-surgical instructions as soon as possible after Dupuytren's contracture surgery in order to promote optimal healing and reduce problems.

Your hand will probably be bandaged or in a splint right after the surgery to protect the incision site and encourage good finger alignment.

Maintaining your hand above the level of your heart is crucial for minimizing edema and enhancing blood flow.

To minimize tension on the surgical site, refrain from engaging in any demanding tasks or heavy lifting with the operated hand.

Hand Therapy And Rehabilitation

Hand therapy and rehabilitation are important components of the healing process following Dupuytren's contracture surgery.

To keep your hands strong and flexible, your doctor might advise you to begin doing stretches and light hand exercises as soon as you can.

Attending hand therapy sessions with a licensed therapist can assist increase functional abilities, decrease stiffness, and improve range of motion.

Various treatments, including massage, manual stretching, and specially designed exercise regimens based on your individual needs, may be included in these sessions.

Handling Soreness And Unease

Following Dupuytren's contracture surgery, pain and discomfort are frequent, but there are a number of effective ways to treat them. Painkillers could be recommended by your doctor to ease your suffering during the early stages of recuperation.

Furthermore, numbness and edema around the surgery site can be lessened by applying ice packs.

It's crucial to adhere to the pain management guidelines provided by your healthcare provider and to get in touch with them if you have severe or ongoing pain that doesn't go away with medicine.

Keeping Complications Like Infection And Recurrence At Bay

Success with Dupuytren's contracture surgery depends on avoiding complications like infection and recurrence. It's critical to adhere to your healthcare provider's instructions for hand treatment and exercises after surgery in order to preserve hand function, prevent contractures from reforming, and reduce the chance of recurrence. Furthermore, maintaining a clean and dry surgical site and using proper hand hygiene might help lower the risk of infection.

For an assessment and course of treatment, get in touch with your healthcare practitioner right away if you observe any indications of infection, such as redness, swelling, or increasing discomfort at the surgical site.

Extended Monitoring And Follow-Up

Monitoring and long-term follow-up are crucial parts of managing Dupuytren's contracture in order to evaluate surgical results and identify possible issues early on.

Regular follow-up appointments will be arranged by your healthcare physician to assess the status of your rehabilitation, track hand function, and handle any potential concerns or problems.

Your healthcare provider may do imaging tests, functional assessments, and physical examinations during these visits to make sure your hand is healing and performing at its best.

For the duration of your recuperation, it is imperative that you keep all of your planned follow-up appointments and let your healthcare provider know about any changes or issues.

40

CHAPTER SIX

REPAY AND RESUMMATION

Timetable For Recuperation

The healing process for Dupuytren's contracture usually has a schedule, regardless of whether it is treated surgically or non-surgically with injections or therapy.

It's crucial to remember that each person's experience may differ depending on a number of variables, including general health, the treatment option selected, and the severity of the ailment.

You might have some hand soreness, edema, and stiffness in the early post-treatment phase. This is common and can be controlled with painkillers that your doctor has prescribed and by adhering to any special post-operative instructions that you have been given.

Your hand's function and mobility will probably gradually improve in the first few days to weeks after treatment.

If your doctor has prescribed physical therapy exercises, they will be very important at this time to promote flexibility and avoid stiffness.

Your hand's strength and range of motion will continue to improve as you move through the healing process, which usually takes several weeks to months.

It's crucial to keep in mind, though, that a full recovery could take many months, and that patience is essential throughout this time.

Improvement In Hand Function Gradually

One common occurrence during the recovery phase is a progressive increase in hand function. Over time, as long as you constantly perform rehabilitation exercises and adhere to your healthcare provider's advice, you should notice a gradual improvement at first.

Regaining optimal hand function, which includes the capacity to hold things, carry out daily duties with ease, and go back to work or other enjoyable activities, is one of the main objectives of rehabilitation.

Exercises for dexterity, strengthening, and stretching that are customized for your needs may be included in this.

It is crucial to approach the healing process with perseverance and patience, realizing that progress might not always be straight-line. Even though you might occasionally hit a roadblock or plateau in your rehabilitation, you can still make progress in your goal of restoring hand function if you're committed to it and persistent.

The Value Of Following Rehabilitation Exercises

Following treatment for Dupuytren's contracture, adherence to rehabilitation exercises is essential for optimizing healing results and avoiding problems. Your physical therapist or healthcare practitioner will probably recommend a customized workout regimen made to meet your unique demands and objectives.

When it comes to rehabilitative activities, consistency is essential. Try to follow your healthcare provider's suggested instructions for frequency and duration when performing the exercises on a regular basis. This could be doing regular strengthening and stretching exercises as well as practicing functional movements that resemble everyday tasks.

Through dedication to your rehabilitation regimen, you can enhance the general function, strength, and flexibility of your hands. Furthermore, maintaining your range of motion and preventing stiffness in your hand joints can be achieved by staying active, which can improve long-term results.

Picking Up Daily Tasks And Work

You will gradually regain the capacity to carry out everyday tasks and, if necessary, return to work as you move through the healing process. The length of time it takes to resume these activities, however, will vary based on a number of variables, including the kind of therapy you had, the nature of your work, and your healthcare provider's advice.

It's critical to be transparent with your healthcare team about your fears and aspirations for going back to work or other activities. They can offer advice on whether it's safe to take up particular activities again as well as methods for adapting activities to account for any residual discomfort or limits.

Restarting work may require modifying your workstation or job responsibilities to account for any lingering symptoms or limitations in hand function. It's possible that your company can offer adjustments or help to make the process of going back to work easier.

Psychological Assistance Throughout The Healing Process

Physically and psychologically taxing, recovery from Dupuytren's contracture can be a long process. It's normal to feel frustrated, anxious, or depressed at this time. It's crucial to put your mental and emotional health first during your rehabilitation process because of this.

During trying times, asking for help from friends, family, or support groups can be quite beneficial in terms of offering emotional support and encouragement.

If you're finding it difficult to handle the difficulties of rehabilitation, you might also think about speaking with a mental health expert.

Additional forms of psychological assistance include education and information about your problem and available treatments. By being aware of what to anticipate during the healing process, you can reduce anxiety and feel more empowered to actively participate in your own care.

Keep in mind that you are not experiencing your recovery alone. Seek advice and assistance from your healthcare team and other accessible resources as you work through the psychological and physical aspects of recovering from Dupuytren's contracture.

CHAPTER SEVEN

MANAGING DUPUYTREN'S CONTRACTURE: COPING MECHANISMS

Managing Physical Restrictions

Although Dupuytren's Contracture imposes physical limits, there are techniques to help manage daily activities more successfully. Setting priorities and dividing work into doable chunks is crucial.

For example, adaptive grips, ergonomic cutlery, and jar openers are examples of assistive equipment that can help reduce hand strain when handling objects. Tasks can also be made easier to do by rearranging commonly used things in your workspace so they are conveniently located.

Asking Friends And Family For Support

Having friends and family support can be very beneficial when managing Dupuytren's Contracture.

Be honest with your loved ones about your needs and limitations, and don't be afraid to ask for help when you need it. In addition to offering emotional support and assistance with difficult activities, friends and relatives can go with you to doctor's appointments.

Recall that receiving assistance from others can make the road less difficult if you are dealing with Dupuytren's Contracture alone.

Taking Part In Online Communities And Support Groups

Getting involved in Dupuytren's Contracture support groups or online forums can help one feel understood and like they belong. These groups provide a forum for exchanging coping mechanisms, experiences, and emotional support.

Getting involved with people who are going through similar things can make you feel less alone and more capable of navigating life with Dupuytren's Contracture.

Additionally, talking to people who have experienced the issue directly may provide you with insightful information about treatment options and lifestyle modifications.

Tools And Adaptive Devices For Everyday Tasks

People with Dupuytren's Contracture can greatly improve their independence and quality of life with the use of adaptive tools and technologies.

If your hand mobility is restricted, think about employing items like dressing aids, buttonhooks, or reachers that are made to fit such needs.

Daily duties like getting dressed, taking care of oneself, and cooking might become easier and less stressful with the help of these devices. Based on your unique needs and abilities, occupational therapists can offer suggestions and help on the best adaptive gadget selection.

Adopting A Positive Attitude And Mindset

Your ability to manage Dupuytren's Contracture can be greatly impacted by keeping an optimistic outlook.

Even though managing a chronic illness might be difficult, you can enhance your general well-being by finding delight in routine tasks and concentrating on the things you can manage. Engage in activities that make you happy and practice self-care practices like mindfulness and relaxation.

Remind yourself to appreciate your accomplishments, no matter how minor they may appear, and surround yourself with encouraging and happy people. You may face life with Dupuytren's Contracture with perseverance and positivity if you adopt an optimistic outlook.

CHAPTER EIGHT

FAQS AND REGULAR QUESTIONS

Is It Possible To Avoid Dupuytren's Contracture?

Because the precise origin of Dupuytren's contracture is unknown, prevention is difficult. However, a number of risk factors, including age, genetics, and specific lifestyle choices, raise the chance of contracting the illness. Although it might not be totally avoidable, there are things you can do to lessen your chance or postpone its commencement.

It's vital to keep up a healthy lifestyle. Sustaining a healthy weight, quitting smoking, and engaging in regular exercise can all improve general hand health. Furthermore, avoiding hand tasks that require trauma or repetitive clutching will assist lessen hand strain and possibly reduce the chance of developing Dupuytren's contracture.

Maintaining flexibility and preventing the development of severe contractures can also be achieved by routinely stretching and exercising the hands and fingers. In this context, hand exercises recommended by a medical practitioner or occupational therapist may be helpful.

It is imperative to address any underlying medical disorders, such as diabetes or alcoholism, that may exacerbate Dupuytren's contracture. Reducing the chance of developing hand contractures can be accomplished by managing these disorders.

Frequent visits to the doctor can also aid in the early detection of Dupuytren's contracture, enabling timely treatment and intervention.

Does Dupuytren's Contracture Run In Families?

Indeed, a sizable hereditary component contributes to Dupuytren's contracture. Those who have a family history of the illness are more likely to get it themselves. Although the precise inheritance pattern is complicated and poorly known, several genes are thought to be involved.

Not everyone with a family history of Dupuytren's contracture will experience the ailment, even if genetics plays a big part. Similarly, some people may get the illness without any family history.

It is imperative that you discuss your family history with your healthcare professional, particularly if you observe any early symptoms or indicators of Dupuytren's contracture. More effective management of the illness can be achieved with early recognition and intervention.

What Is The Likelihood Of A Recurrence Following Surgery?

The severity of the ailment, the kind of surgery done, and the individual healing factors all influence the chance of recurrence following Dupuytren's contracture surgery.

In general, the risk of recurrence increases with the severity of the contracture and the aggressiveness of the surgery needed to treat it. Furthermore, a family history of Dupuytren's contracture and other conditions including diabetes and smoking may raise the chance of recurrence.

Recurrence rates can vary greatly, based on the patient population and study, from approximately 5% to 65%. Before undertaking any surgical therapy for Dupuytren's contracture, it is imperative to have a discussion with your surgeon regarding the possibility of recurrence.

To address recurrence, additional treatments or procedures including collagenase injections, radiation therapy, or repeat surgery can be required in some circumstances. The best course of action for you will depend on your unique situation, which your healthcare professional can help determine.

Can Altering One's Lifestyle Aid In Managing The Illness?

Although modifying one's lifestyle may not be enough to cure Dupuytren's contracture, it can assist in controlling symptoms and possibly decrease the condition's progression. Changes in lifestyle that could be advantageous include:

Giving up smoking:

Research has shown that smoking increases the risk of Dupuytren's contracture and exacerbates symptoms. Giving up smoking can help delay the onset of the illness and enhance general hand health.

Sustaining An Appropriate Weight:

Obesity or being overweight can exacerbate Dupuytren's contracture by putting more strain on the hands and joints. Reducing this stress can be accomplished by eating right and exercising to maintain a healthy weight.

Steer clear of repetitive hand trauma: Hand trauma or repetitive gripping activities can aggravate pre-existing Dupuytren's contracture symptoms or raise the chance of acquiring new ones. Hand strain can be lessened by using caution when using your hands and by pausing when necessary.

• Frequent exercise: Maintaining range of motion and flexibility in the hands and fingers through gentle stretching and exercise may help lessen the severity of contractures. A healthcare provider's recommended hand exercises or occupational therapy may be helpful.

It is imperative that you address any changes in lifestyle with your healthcare provider, who may offer tailored advice depending on your unique situation and the degree of your Dupuytren's contracture.

Where can I locate trustworthy sources and assistance regarding Dupuytren's Contracture?

Navigating treatment choices and managing Dupuytren's contracture can be greatly aided by finding trustworthy resources and support. Here are a few locations to begin:

Healthcare providers: You can get important information about Dupuytren's contracture, including diagnosis, treatment choices, and ongoing management, from your primary care physician or a hand specialist.

Patient advocacy groups: For those impacted by Dupuytren's contracture, groups like the Dupuytren Foundation and the International Dupuytren Society provide information, tools, and support. These groups might include training guides, discussion boards, and chances to meet people going through comparable difficulties.

Online resources: People can access information, communicate with others, and exchange experiences on a number of websites and online forums devoted to Dupuytren's contracture. It is imperative, nevertheless, to be certain that the data originates from reliable sources and to confirm any information with a medical expert.

Support groups: Joining a group for people with Dupuytren's contracture can offer motivation, encouragement, and practical assistance in addition to emotional support. Support groups are a great tool for people coping with the difficulties of having Dupuytren's contracture; they can meet in person or virtually.

People who are impacted by Dupuytren's contracture can find helpful information, support, and the ability to take charge of their condition by making use of these resources and support networks.

www.ingramcontent.com/pod-product-compliance
Lightning Source LLC
Chambersburg PA
CBHW071843210526
45479CB00001B/270